Top Daily Practices to Lose Weight Quickly:

The Best Methods for Permanent Weight Loss

Mary E. Nelson

Table of contents

Chapter 1: One small activity at a time will help you lose weight.

It may seem like you're on an uphill, downhill roller coaster while trying to lose weight. Adopt a few little, simple habits to assist you in moving toward a more solid footing.

You will continue to advance in the direction of your objective as your small habits develop into larger ones that can significantly change how you behave.

Winning Techniques
Small behavioral changes may be helpful since you can succeed quickly. Every time you maintain a small behavior, your confidence increases. You feel like you have more power.

If you've developed a certain tiny habit, you can also lessen anxiety about whether you're doing "it right" or doing "enough." You can record it as a success each time you stick to your small habit, such as eating a vegetable every day for lunch.

Less is more.
The most important consideration when choosing a little habit is making it something you can do. Prepare yourself to succeed.

With time, you may strengthen that simple habit for even better results. For instance, once eating a vegetable every day at lunch becomes second nature, you can go on to the next stage of your goal. That might entail serving your daily evening meal with two vegetables.

Making little habits has the benefit of allowing you to adopt others after one becomes usual. By taking modest efforts, you continue to move forward steadily toward a substantial transformation.

Connect your motivator to the habit. Because it takes effort to stop bad habits, you need a strong justification for starting a new one.

The desire to get healthier is a great reason to do something. If that inspires you, fantastic! If it doesn't, try picking something more straightforward and explicit.

Use the money you would have spent on soda to reward yourself with something special as a way to get yourself to drink water instead of soda. modern music? a special magazine?

Your emotions or thoughts may also play a bigger role in your motivation. You might feel healthier and more natural if you drink water.

Create a trigger to act as a prompt for what has to be done. A trigger may be thought of as an adverse event that causes you to behave badly. For instance, someone may overeat as a result of sadness. But a trigger can also be useful.

A trigger could act as a prompt to engage in your favored habit. It may only be necessary to set an alarm or pick a good spot to post a note.

You need a trigger that will be noticeable to you, ideally at the habit's scheduled time. You may, for instance, take these steps to remind yourself to drink water:

Set a time on your calendar for when you will "meet" with a glass of water.
Connect your habit to routine activities. Remind yourself to drink water by using the process of turning on the water to wash your hands.

Keep going and going
You might occasionally feel less motivated to accomplish your goal, even if you have a clear, attainable goal, strong motivation, and a trigger that reminds you to carry out your small habit. When that occurs, it's time to assemble more assistance.

Support your new actions. Ask a family member or close friend to keep in mind why you are playing the game by explaining what you are doing. At this point, you might choose to use Facebook or another social media site.

Addressing oneself. If you're tempted to skip a workout or eat something you've decided against, simple reminders like "I always feel better after a walk" or "That doughnut is not part of my plan" could help you stay on track.

Weight loss takes time. The small-habit approach won't aid in rapid weight loss. But it can aid in keeping you on track without requiring you to make a huge life adjustment. By adding one small behavior at a time, you can build strong, healthy habits that you can use to keep your weight under control.

Chapter 2: Healthy habits to lose weight

Whether it is healthy or unhealthy behavior, a habit is something you instinctively do. Successful weight loss leads to the development of healthy eating habits.

These healthy eating habits may help you lose weight and keep it off.

Create Your Kitchen
Sweet goods on your kitchen's shelves may promote unhealthy eating behaviors. Rearrange your kitchen so that nutrient-dense foods are the default option.

Always consume nutritious food. Keep a plate of fruit on the counter and pre-cut vegetables in the refrigerator. You'll always have a healthy snack available for times when you're hungry.
reduce the urge to indulge. If you know you can't control yourself around cookies or other

diet-busting foods, keep them out of your reach or, even better, leave the house.

Eat with utensils at all times. Eating straight from a container or bag promotes overeating.

Use smaller plates. If you start a meal with less food in front of you, you'll likely consume less overall.

Eat a More Balanced Diet

Since life gets busy, a lot of individuals eat without thinking about what they're putting in their mouths. By implementing the following habits, you can stop this mindless eating.

Eat your breakfast. Overeating is a call of the hungry stomach. A piece of fruit, whole-grain bread or cereal, low-fat milk, or yogurt is a good way to start the day.

Plan ahead. Before you get hungry, decide what you're going to eat. Once you're content, make a plan for your meals and begin your buying. The capacity to reject unhealthy options will rise.

Turn off the television. When you are utilizing a computer, TV, or another distracting screen, your focus is taken away from what you are eating. If you aren't allowed to taste your food, you are more likely to overeat.

Consume healthy foods first. If you start the meal with soup or a salad, you'll feel less hungry when you go on to the main course. Simply avoid cream-based soups and salad dressings that are high in calories.

Frequently consume fast snacks. Instead of two or three large meals, you might spread out your meals throughout the day to keep yourself full.

Verify your weight. The information from the scale can help you figure out how your eating habits affect your weight.

Ensure that your house is cool. Feeling a little chilly throughout the winter may help you burn more calories than keeping your home on the warm side.

Eliminate bad behaviors

Emotional eating, which is often referred to as eating for comfort rather than nutrition, can have a big impact on what and how much you eat. To alter your relationship with food:

Be careful. Pay attention to the effects of different foods on your body. Maybe right now, fried food tastes amazing. How will it feel in your stomach, though, in an hour?
Hurry up. Place your fork down or start a conversation in between bites. Pacing oneself gives your stomach a chance to experience fullness.
Note this. Verify the nutrient content of an item before consuming it. List the foods you intend to eat before you begin. Both of these behaviors make you pause before swallowing so that you can think them through.

Change the way you talk about food. Instead of saying "I can't eat it," say "I don't eat that." You can feel cheated if you refuse. You take the initiative when you claim that you don't.
Obtain Guidance
Your family and friends can encourage you and help you stay motivated. Select a company that

understands how crucial this is and that will support you rather than criticize or tempt you with their poor habits.

Chapter 3: How fruits and veggies can aid with weight management.

Increasing your intake of fruits, vegetables, whole grains, lean meats, nuts, and legumes is a simple way to lose weight or keep it off. A diet rich in fruits and vegetables may also reduce your risk of contracting certain malignancies and other chronic diseases. In addition, fruits and vegetables include essential vitamins, minerals, fiber, and other nutrients for good health.

To lose weight, you must consume fewer calories than your body requires.
This does not necessarily mean that you should eat less. You may make lower-calorie versions of some of your favorite foods by substituting low-calorie fruits and vegetables for ingredients with higher calories. With their water and fiber, fruits and vegetables add volume to your meals, enabling you to eat the same amount of food

while ingesting fewer calories. In general, fruits and vegetables are satiating and naturally low in calories and fat.

Simple methods to save calories and increase intake of fruits and vegetables each day
A Healthy Start to the Day at Breakfast
Change one egg or half the cheese in your breakfast omelet with spinach, onions, or mushrooms. Vegetables add greater volume and flavor to the meal while having fewer calories than an egg or a slice of cheese.
Reduce the amount of cereal in your bowl to create room for some half-sliced banana, peach, or strawberry slices. The food is still edible in its entirety, but there are fewer calories.

Change the 2 ounces of cheese and 2 ounces of meat in your sandwich, wrap, or burrito with vegetables like lettuce, tomatoes, cucumbers, or onions. The new version contains fewer calories than the previous one.

Replace 2 ounces of meat or 1 cup of noodles in a broth-based soup with 1 cup of finely chopped vegetables, such as broccoli, carrots, beans, or red peppers. After eating the vegetables, you'll be full and won't feel the need for additional calories.

Replace the rice or pasta in your favorite recipe with 1 cup of chopped vegetables, such as broccoli, tomatoes, squash, onions, or peppers. The dish with the vegetables will still be extremely full even if it has the same number of calories as the original dish.

Take a close look at your serving dish. Vegetables, fruit, and whole grains should make up the majority of your plate. If they don't, you can replace some of the meat, cheese, white pasta, or rice with beans, steamed broccoli, asparagus, greens, or another favorite vegetable. This will allow you to reduce the number of calories in your meal without reducing the amount of food you eat. But remember to use a small or ordinary plate rather than a platter. The total number of calories you consume is still important even if a substantial percentage of them come from fruits and vegetables.

wholesome snacks

Most healthy eating plans allow one or two small snacks per day. By choosing mostly fruits and vegetables, you can have a snack that has only 100 calories.

A medium-sized apple has 100 calories or fewer (72 calories)

a typical banana

1 cup of steamed blueberries, 1 cup of grapes, and 1 cup of green beans.

1 cup of carrots, bell peppers, or broccoli (30 calories each), along with 2 tablespoons of hummus

Instead of buying a high-calorie snack from the vending machine, bring some cut-up fruit or vegetables from home. A 1-ounce bag of corn chips has the same number of calories as a small apple, a cup of whole strawberries, and a cup of carrots with 1/4 cup of low-calorie dip combined. If you pick one or two of these substitutes for the chips, you can have a satisfying snack with fewer calories.

Recall that substitution is the essential element.
fruit and vegetable picture
Fruits and vegetables nevertheless contain calories, although having fewer than many other foods. If you start eating fruits and vegetables in addition to what you normally consume, you will be adding calories and running the danger of gaining weight. Replacement is the key. Eat fruits and vegetables rather than other high-calorie items.

Eat fruits and vegetables as they were designed to be eaten or prepare them in a low-fat or fat-free way.
Consider steaming your vegetables, using low-calorie or low-fat components in the dressing, and adding herbs and spices for taste. When a dish is prepared using particular techniques, such as breading and frying, or when high-fat dressings or sauces are used, the number of calories and fat in the dish will be greatly

increased. Eat the fruit raw to feel its natural sweetness.

Canned or frozen fruits and veggies are also fantastic options.
The nutrients in canned or frozen fruits and vegetables can match those in their fresh counterparts. It is best to choose those without added sugar, syrup, cream sauces, or other high-calorie ingredients.

Choose whole fruit over fruit juices and drinks. Fruit juices are devoid of the fiber found in actual fruit.
It is recommended to do this because the whole fruit has extra fiber that increases feelings of fullness. In comparison to the 85 calories in a 6-ounce portion of orange juice, a medium orange has only 65 calories.

Fruit that is dried provides a larger snack for the same number of calories than fruit that is whole.

A small box of raisins contains roughly 100 calories (1/4 cup). For the same number of calories, you may have 1 cup of grapes.

Chapter 4: Healthy diet for rapid weight loss

To reduce weight, you don't have to deprive yourself.

The key to healthy eating is understanding what foods to eat and avoid, as well as those that may cause your insulin levels to surge. It's not that difficult to lose tons of weight or discover the secret to hormonal balance while meeting all of your nutritional needs. When you believe you've got the answers, a brand-new idea will make you question what you were just so certain about. Here is a meal plan that will help you lose weight without drastically reducing your calorie intake.

"Keeping fit involves learning about your body constantly, adjusting your diet and exercise regimen as necessary, and making sure your health is as good as it can be. Healthy food is usually simple to prepare. Eating food that has been lightly cooked and avoid combining too many food types is key.

You'll soon reach your fitness objectives if you follow this diet plan for losing weight:
1. Make informed dietary decisions
No more than one protein category (dairy, meats, eggs, dals, legumes, pulses, tofu), one carb group (rice, millet, wheat), and one or two servings of vegetables should be included in any of your main meals, such as breakfast, lunch, or dinner.

"By better activating the enzymes, keeping your combinations simple will allow for easier digestion. Keeping the combos inexpensive will also make it possible for you to eat in moderation. The more options you have, the more you'll likely consume because the palate loves variety.

2. Timing is crucial

Maintain consistent mealtimes throughout the day. You manage your appetite better, have fewer cravings, and go about your day without ghrelin, the hunger hormone, rising. A fat-storage hormone, ghrelin. The fewer times it rears its head, the easier it will be to control your eating habits and cravings. The secret is to avoid getting hungry during the day, eat every two to three hours, and eat 20 minutes before you anticipate getting hungry. And observe how pleasantly you will be able to control your portions, scales, and hunger.

3. Stay hydrated.

Drink warm or cold water when you're hungry. It is common to confuse hunger and thirst.

4. Light meals work "Keep your meals light two nights a week by having just a soup and a salad with fresh raw, stir-fried vegetables garnished with 5-10 grams of nuts and, if necessary, a serving of whole-grain carbohydrates like wheat, brown rice, or amaranth.

5. Spread out your mealtimes.
Keep a 12-hour window clear of food and liquids between the time you finish dinner and the start of breakfast. Five days a week, given that.

6. Continue to enjoy indulgent meals.
Menon recommends, "Whether it's the weekends or not, give your body a cheerful boost by indulging in whatever it craves! The richness of a moderate amount of butter or ghee can be used to make cheat meals like sweets or fried pleasure, an excess of carbohydrates, or the meats you love so much. Your hormones of happiness will increase, and you will too.

Chapter 5: How Snacking Can Aid with Weight Loss

Many of us frequently consider eliminating snacks from our diets when trying to reduce weight. It sounds like a sensible method to regulate your metabolism and cut out on fat- and calorie-dense foods in your diet. Snacking wisely on the proper meals, however, can aid in weight loss.

You can truly balance your diet and avoid overeating at meals with a few easy, healthy adjustments. We tend to overeat when we skip snacks since it makes us feel more hungry before meals. Here are three suggestions for developing a snacking routine that can sate your hunger and help you lose weight.

Organizing Snacks to Maintain Focus

Always follow a timetable if you want your diet to be successful. Include daily snacks in your eating plan. This makes it easier for you to estimate your calorie and other dietary intakes. Additionally, since your body is breaking down food more frequently when you snack, it can increase your metabolism. You can lose weight more quickly by including snacks in your diet plan, provided the food is balanced and healthy.

Try to eat every three to four hours.

Once it has been four hours since your last meal or snack, blood sugar levels begin to fall. Make sure you eat every three to four hours to maintain your body on a more effective digestive schedule to prevent this. To allow for adequate digestion, it's also crucial to wait at least 30 minutes after your last meal before going to bed.

Avoid packaged foods, low-fat products, and "light" foods.

Along with having negative impacts on your weight, packaged meals and low-fat snacks include hazardous chemicals that can lead to cancer and heart disease, among other health issues. These foods typically contain a lot of sugar, and 'light' ones often have extra sodium to make up for the blandness. Choose healthy snacks only, such as fresh fruit or nuts. Try to eliminate packaged foods from your diet altogether, excluding just when you're snacking. To increase your daily food consumption, look for natural meats and cereals.

It's critical to pay attention to what you're putting into your body when dieting. Keep a daily food journal and check that you are staying within your daily calorie and fat allowances. Call our office right away for more details on efficient weight loss methods and dieting.

Chapter 6: How Drinking More Water Can Help You Lose Weight

Weight loss has long been associated with drinking water.

In reality, 30–59% of Americans are attempting to use less water.

Numerous studies suggest that drinking more water may aid in weight loss and maintenance.

Water Intake Can Boost Calorie Burn
Most studies looked at what happened when you drank one serving or 0.5 liters (17 oz) of water.

Drinking water increases your resting energy expenditure (REE), also known as calorie expenditure.
Humans have been seen to experience a 24–30% increase in resting energy expenditure within 10

minutes of eating water. At least an hour passes during this.

Drinking cold water raised resting energy expenditure by 25%, according to a study of overweight and obese children.

In a study of obese women, the consequences of consuming more water—more than 1 liter (34 ounces) per day—were examined. They found that doing so resulted in an extra 2 kg (4.4 lbs) of weight loss over a year.

Given that these ladies just upped their water intake, these results are remarkable.

These two studies also found that drinking 0.5 liters (17 oz) of water led to an additional 23 calories being burned. This equates to more than 2 kg (4.4 lbs) of fat or about 17,000 calories each year.

Numerous further studies observed overweight persons who drank 1-1.5 liters (34-50 oz) of water each day over a few weeks. They found significant reductions in body weight, body mass index, waist circumference, and body fat (BMI).

These results can be much more startling when the water is chilly. When you drink cold water, your body uses additional calories to reheat it to body temperature.

Drinking 0.5 liters (17 oz) of water for at least an hour may increase the number of calories burned. Some studies suggest that this could lead to mild weight loss.

Water Can Suppress Hunger Before Meals
Some people claim that drinking water before a meal reduces appetite.

This does seem to have some validity, but primarily among middle-aged and older people.

Studies on older people show that drinking water before each meal can hasten weight loss by 2 kg (4.4 lbs) over 12 weeks.

In one study, middle-aged overweight and obese people who drank water before each meal lost 44% more weight than those who did not.

Another study found that drinking water before breakfast reduced the number of calories consumed during the meal by 13%.

Although this may be quite beneficial for middle-aged and older folks, studies on younger people have not shown the same significant reduction in calorie intake.

Drinking water before meals can help persons in their middle years and older eat less. This reduces calorie consumption, which results in weight loss.

Lower risk of weight gain and lower calorie intake are both related to increased water drinking.

Because water is naturally calorie-free, it is frequently linked to lower calorie intake.

You now prefer drinking water over other, typically sugar- and calorie-rich beverages, which is mostly to blame.

Observational research has shown that people who drink mostly water frequently take in 200 calories (or 9%) fewer calories than the average individual.

Drinking water may also help prevent long-term weight gain. The typical person gains 1.45 kg (3.2 lbs) of weight every four years.
This amount could be reduced by:

Adding 1 cup of water: You might prevent this 0.13 kg weight gain by consuming 1 cup extra water each day (0.23 lbs).
Use water instead of other beverages: 0Over four years, substituting one cup of water for one serving of a sugar-sweetened beverage may prevent a weight gain of 0.5 kg (1.1 lbs).

Water consumption can prevent children from being overweight or obese, thus encour0age youngsters to do so. This is particularly significant.

In a recent study, water drinking among children was encouraged with the goal of reducing obesity rates. They installed water faucets in 17 schools and instructed second and third-graders about water usage in the classroom.

Schools that raised water consumption witnessed a startling 31% reduction in the incidence of obesity after just one academic year.

Particularly in young people, drinking more water may reduce calorie intake, lessen the risk of obesity, and prevent long-term weight gain.

Water Should Be Consumed When?
Many health groups recommend drinking eight 8-ounce glasses (or 2 liters) of water each day.

But this number is random. Like so many other things, how much water a person needs is largely up to them (20).

People who exercise frequently or perspire a lot, for example, can need more water than those who aren't as active.

Elderly people and nursing mothers should both carefully monitor their water intake.

Keep in mind that many foods and beverages, most notably fruits and vegetables, coffee, tea, meat, fish, and milk, also include water.

When you're thirsty, you should always drink water, and you should drink just enough to quench your thirst.

If you have headaches, mood swings, voracious appetite, or problems concentrating, you could be mildly dehydrated. Drinking more water might be beneficial.

Studies show that 1-2 liters of water each day should be sufficient to promote weight loss.

The suggested water intakes in various measures are listed below:

1 to 2 liters.
67 to 34 ounces.
4–8 8-ounce glasses.
However, this is merely a general suggestion. Some could need less, while others might need a lot more.

It's also not a good idea to drink too much water because it can lead to water poisoning. This has even led to death in severe situations, such as water-drinking contests.

According to studies, consuming 1-2 liters of water each day, ideally, before meals, is enough to encourage weight loss.

Weight loss is greatly aided by water.

It has no calories at all, boosts calorie burn, and, when consumed before meals, may even lessen appetite.

The benefits are even greater if you switch from sugary drinks to water. A really easy method exists for cutting back on calories and sugar.

However, keep in mind that drinking water alone won't be enough if you want to shed a significant quantity of weight.

Chapter 7: How Eating Mindfully Can Help You Lose Weight

Most of us have a very clear understanding of the concept of mindless eating. We do it when watching television, working on a computer project, using our phones, and even while we are driving. You can finish a bag of chips or a few cookies without stopping to consider it or even genuinely noticing that you are chewing and swallowing. According to studies, on the other hand, when we focus on what we're eating while eating undisturbed, we develop a healthy relationship with food, may lose more weight and are more likely to keep it off.

"Mindful eating can help reduce the hedonistic need to eat, which is characterized by a lack of self-control, obsession with food, and an unfulfilled sense [independent of physical hunger.] You might appreciate food more when you eat thoughtfully.

Some people might be turned off by the idea of mindful eating because they think it requires meditating for 20 minutes before each meal or that you have to stop and express gratitude for each bite of food.

However, it might only require you to pay attention to what you eat and how you feel while you're eating.

Healthy Eating vs. Dieting
It's general knowledge that shedding pounds only requires willpower. If you can restrain yourself from overeating and resist your cravings, you will lose weight. Traditional diets, however, don't give people the tools they need to control their emotions or deal with cravings, which might lead them to overeat. In this situation, mindful eating is important. You're advised to examine your wants and accept them

for what they are as opposed to attempting to stifle them.

Weight Loss-Friendly Foods

Traditional dieting also places a strong emphasis on limitation, rules, and frequently, judgment. Based on their choice of meals, dieters frequently classify themselves as "good" or "bad" foods. Eating mindfully removes any guilt or value judgments from the food you are consuming. Instead of being told "no, don't eat this," individuals are urged to eat the foods they prefer consciously and without judgment.

Science Behind Mindful Eating

An analysis of research articles that were published in the journal Nutrition Research Reviews in 2017 found that mindful-eating therapies were the most effective in treating binge eating, emotional eating, and eating in response to outside cues. It might be easier to alter such ingrained eating habits if you practice mindful eating, which has the potential to "rewire" your brain in some way. One researcher who employs neurofeedback devices on patients claims, "We can observe that the area of the brain that gets stimulated when we're caught up in cravings and emotional eating is inhibited when we're being mindful."

Weight loss typically occurs as a result of a shift in eating habits. As an illustration, in a 2018 study that was published in the Journal of Family Medicine & Community Health, researchers looked into the potential effects that a 15-week weight-reduction program with mindful-eating techniques would have on eating patterns and weight loss. The total number of participants was divided into two groups, one of which received the intervention, and the other served as the control group. Those in the intervention group lost weight six times faster than participants in the control group did. Ninety-eight percent of the mindful eating group reported continuing their habits after a six-month check-up.
Increasing people's awareness of the food they eat is a powerful habit-changing tactic.

According to studies, mindful eating offers benefits even if weight loss is not achieved. In a 2016 study of 194 obese adults, it was discovered that those who got mindfulness training in addition to diet and exercise advice saw significantly lower fasting blood glucose and cholesterol levels than the group who only received advice on healthy eating and physical activity. According to research, the mindful eating group cut back on sweets throughout the intervention and continued to do so even six months later, which is what caused the health improvements.

How to Eat Mindfully

The core of mindful eating is paying more attention to your hunger, cravings, food, and how your body feels before, during, and after eating. When you sit down for your next meal, try putting some of these simple strategies into practice.

• Assess your hunger (and then assess it again). Being aware of your physical hunger is one of the keys to mindful eating. Before you eat, rank your level of hunger on a scale of 1 to 10. Once you've had a few nibbles, ask again. As the meal progresses, switch to evaluating your level of satiety on a scale of 1 to 10. Aim to stop eating when you are moderately full, or about a 7, to help prevent overeating.

• Take it easy. You may enjoy each meal more and keep track of your satiety levels if you eat more slowly. Therefore, it should not come as a surprise that a recent six-year study involving about 60,000 people discovered that those who went from rapid to leisurely eating experienced a 42 percent lower rate of obesity than those who did the opposite.

• Maintain your focus. Mindless overeating may happen from any activity that keeps you from paying attention to your meals, such as watching television, using social media, reading, or even participating in an interesting conversation.

• Recognize your desires. It's better to let yourself experience hunger than to try to talk yourself out of it. Simply explained, cravings are physical feelings that grow stronger the more we try to ignore or avoid them. Instead of trying to suppress the impulse, focus on how it affects your body's sensations, think about what might be triggering it, and even spend some time tasting and admiring the food you're craving. After a few deep breaths of calmness, take another look to see if it still catches your attention.

• Savor the first tastes. Even if you're paying attention, if you decide that you do want to eat something, go ahead. However, eat it slowly, attentively, and savor each bite. According to a study, the majority of satisfaction is experienced during the first few bites of a beloved food. If you take the time to focus on the sensory sensation of those first bites, you could find that your hunger is satiated without overindulging.

Chapter 8: How to Monitor Your Food for Weight Loss

Numerous diet and exercise fads claim that they might help you lose a lot of weight quickly. Even though many fads fail when it comes to keeping weight off, this is the area where success lies. The key to attaining long-lasting weight loss may be as simple as tracking your food intake, also referred to as "dietary self-management." It's important to start here because it's straightforward and will help you lose weight.

Simply, if you consume more calories than you burn off, you will gain weight. On the other side, if you burn more calories than you consume, you will lose weight. Of course, there are many factors at work here, such as hormones, hydration, and stress, so the concept is not that straightforward.

But you need to make a calorie deficit if you want to lose weight. This suggests that to lose weight, you should focus on burning more calories than you consume.

How can your diet be monitored to help you lose weight?
There are various strategies to monitor your food consumption for weight loss. There are several ways to track eating. Utilizing smartphone applications with barcode scanners and other features to simplify the process is the most widely used option. When utilizing an app to begin or maintain weight loss, take consistency and frequency into account.

Keeping a consistent food journal for more than three days a week may aid in weight loss.

You can track your macros—the proportion of carbohydrates, protein, and fat—in a mobile nutrition app, as well as your calorie or point intake. Please be advised that some of the calories listed in these applications are estimates and may not match what you are eating. You cannot rely on these applications to provide precise measurements, even though they can be useful and motivating tools for your weight loss journey.

Some people may find more success with a more detailed food diary or journal, particularly those who have struggled with their weight for a long time. If you are more interested in gaining a general understanding of your eating habits and trends but are not particularly interested in data analysis, a food diary or log may be a suitable tool for tracking your diet for weight loss.

What to include in your food diary
Start by following the fundamentals of weight-loss nutrition. Use a food scale, measuring cups, and measuring spoons when preparing your food. This holds regardless of whether you use an app or a food diary. In contrast, people usually underestimate their consumption when evaluating measures or

remembering a past meal, making it impossible to adequately track their intake.

Whatever method you use to keep track of your meals, be as descriptive as you can about how they were prepared, how much you consumed, and the precise ingredients of each dish.

You must be quite selective while choosing your diet foods. Simply logging chicken, for instance, is insufficient; you also need to specify whether it was skinless, produced with light flesh, organ meat or was baked or fried. If you had a salad, mention how much dressing was used. Indicate whether cheese or nuts were added in addition to the specified amount.

To ensure optimal nutrition for weight loss, you must be conscious of how and when you are weighing or measuring the items you eat. As an illustration, the nutritional value of foods like pasta and rice is often given on the packaging in terms of weight before cooking. Therefore, you would need to measure them before cooking. As a bonus, 100g of cooked chicken might include 165 calories and 31g of protein as opposed to 115 calories and 23g of protein in 100g of raw chicken. This might not seem like a big difference. However, even a little underestimate of the calories in the food over time might add up.

You might also consider maintaining a journal of your appetite. Think about whether you ate because you were hungry or to get away from work. Before a meal, you can jot down your emotions and ideas. Consider if you ate the cake out of stress and distress or whether you actively decided to treat yourself and then relished every bite. Finally, make a note of where you were when you ate the cake and who you were with.

Your food journal may have columns that include the following data:

Time
Food Amount (or calories)
Hunger Level Location

Who were you with?

benefits of keeping a food journal

Food tracking's primary objectives are accountability and promoting awareness. Even though it might seem simple, breathing before eating has many advantages. An effective meal-tracking system can help you keep track of what you eat. You can then record the food in your food journal before eating it. This technique makes you more accountable to yourself and your goals.

Additionally, food tracking helps you address problem areas and build on your strengths by revealing your behaviors. Recognizing, celebrating, and rewarding healthy habits can be just as effective as focusing on the ones you want to change.

You can identify patterns and triggers that are sabotaging your weight loss efforts by keeping note of when, when, and with whom you consume. The first step in changing your behavior is identifying your routines and triggers, whether they be a friend who always orders fast food or a stressful meeting that impairs judgment.

What can you do after recording your food-related data?
Keep reviewing your meal journal regularly since you can discover some fascinating patterns there. For instance, you might find that you miss lunch on days when things are busy or reach for unhealthy foods in the late afternoon, which causes you to overeat later. A critical first step in modifying your behavior is identifying these issue areas and developing ways to deal with them.

You can also find that some foods increase mood or give you more energy. If there are advantages to consuming particular foods, it would be easier to stick to your dietary plan. After all, realizing that eating well helps you feel better might motivate you to do it more often.

Keeping track of your intake allows you to look back and evaluate your diet. After a few weeks of routinely keeping track of your meals, take some time to consider the following:

Which type of diet do I follow?
Do I consume a sufficient amount and variety of fruits and vegetables?
Do I eat enough whole grains in my diet?
Am I choosing lean sources of protein?
Do I consume healthy fats?
How do my eating habits and how I feel influence each other?
Can I spot any trends or develop any unhealthy habits?
Can I change my habits to make weight loss easier?
What can I do, in the simplest way, to change my diet?
What actions can I do right away to make better decisions?
What can I infer about eating well from that particular day?

By giving open and honest answers to these questions, it might be able to reach and maintain a healthy weight.

Chapter 9: Sleep and Weight Loss

Losing weight can be difficult, and maintaining weight loss can be even more difficult. Even though the medical community is still working to grasp the nuanced relationship between sleep and body weight, several apparent correlations have emerged that highlight the possible weight loss benefits of getting a full night's rest and the harmful health impacts of sleep deprivation.

Weight Gain and Sleep: A Relationship
Over the past few decades[1], both the length of time Americans spend sleeping and the perceived quality of their sleep have decreased. During a significant chunk of the same period, the average body mass index (BMI) of Americans increased[2], indicating a trend toward higher body weights and elevated rates of obesity.

In response to these modifications, numerous research began to examine potential connections between weight and sleep. Numerous studies have found a connection between sleep deprivation and poor sleep quality and metabolic irregularities, weight gain, an elevated risk of obesity, and other long-term health issues.

The exact nature of this association is still a subject of debate among medical experts, but the research that is currently in hand points to a connection between restful sleep and healthy body weight.

Most of the subtleties of the connection between sleep and weight remain unknown. Several theories suggest lines of inquiry for additional research to improve our understanding of the relationship between sleep and weight and preventing obesity.

Can Lack Sleep Increase Appetite?
One widely accepted view on the connection between sleep and weight is that sleep affects

appetite. Contrary to popular belief, which holds that hunger is solely a function of the stomach growling, hunger is regulated by neurotransmitters, which are chemical messengers that enable neurons (nerve cells) to communicate with one another.

Leptin and ghrelin neurotransmitters are thought to be important for hunger. Ghrelin makes people feel hungry, whereas leptin aids in feeling full. These neurotransmitters' levels in the body typically change during the day, indicating a need for food that contains calories.

Lack of sleep may affect how these neurotransmitters are controlled by the body. One study found that compared to males who slept for 10 hours, men who slept for 4 hours had greater ghrelin levels and lower leptin levels. This imbalance of ghrelin and leptin in sleep-deprived people may lead to an increase in appetite and a decrease in feelings of fullness.

Additionally, several studies have demonstrated that a lack of sleep affects food habits. People who don't get enough sleep often choose foods that are high in calories and carbs.

Two more hypotheses explaining the connection between sleep and increased hunger are the body's endocannabinoid system and orexin6, a neurotransmitter that numerous sleep treatments target.

Numerous researchers believe that additional studies are necessary to completely comprehend the neurobiological relationship between sleep problems and neurotransmitter dysregulation.

Does Sleep Increase Metabolism?
Metabolism is the physiological process by which the body converts the food and liquids we consume into the energy we need to exist. Every single one of our collective activities—including breathing, exercising, and everything in between—is a part of the metabolism. Exercise and other activities can temporarily increase

metabolism, but sleep cannot. The morning is when metabolism is at its lowest because it drops by 15% while we sleep.

Numerous studies have shown that sleep deprivation, which can be caused by self-induction, insomnia, untreated sleep apnea, or other sleep problems, frequently leads to metabolic dysregulation. Poor sleep is associated with elevated oxidative stress, glucose intolerance (a condition that can result in diabetes), and insulin resistance. More eating opportunities may arise from being awake longer, and losing sleep may disrupt your circadian cycles and result in weight gain.

How do sleep and exercise go together?
You can have less energy for exercise and physical activity if you lose sleep. Sports and exercise, particularly weightlifting and balance exercises, can be riskier when you're weary. Even though scientists are still working to fully understand this relationship, exercise is essential to maintaining weight loss and overall health.

Regular exercise, especially if it involves exposure to natural light, can improve the quality of sleep. Even a quick walk during the day may improve sleep, but more vigorous activity may have a more noticeable impact. By engaging in moderate to vigorous exercise for at least 150 minutes per week, one can improve daily attention and minimize daytime sleepiness.

Sleep and Obesity
Inadequate sleep is generally recognized to raise the risk of obesity in children and adolescents, and the precise reason for this link is still up for debate. In addition to the metabolic anomalies we previously discussed, children who don't get enough sleep may skip breakfast in the morning and eat more starchy, sugary, salty, and fatty foods.

Research on adults is less well understood. Although it is challenging for this study to prove a cause-and-effect relationship, a thorough review of previous data shows that those who get less than 6 hours of sleep per night are more likely to be classified as obese. Obesity may increase the prevalence of two disorders: depression and sleep apnea. In this research, it's not apparent whether getting less sleep promotes obesity, whether obesity causes people to get less sleep, or whether the two factors interact. Although more investigation is necessary to completely comprehend this connection, doctors suggest improving sleep quality to combat adult obesity.

Losing Weight While Sleeping
Get enough, quality sleep as part of a healthy weight loss regimen. Most significantly, research has shown that skipping sleep while on a diet might result in slower weight loss and encourage overeating.

The Best Ways to Sleep Well While Losing Weight
There are numerous methods for improving sleep. Here are a few tips that have been proven

to work for improving sleep quality while dieting:

Keep a consistent sleeping routine. Your metabolism can be affected by abrupt changes in your sleep schedule or trying to catch up on sleep after a week of late nights, which makes it simpler for your blood sugar to rise.
Sleep in a room with low light. Exposure to artificial light while sleeping, such as that from a TV or bedside lamp, has been associated with a higher risk of weight gain and obesity.

Don't eat right before bed: Your attempts to lose weight may be hampered if you eat late at night.
Reduce Stress: One way that persistent stress can lead to restless nights and weight gain is by eating to cope with unpleasant feelings.
Being an early bird will help you avoid gaining weight because those who stay up later tend to eat more calories. Early risers may have a better chance of keeping off weight loss than night owls.

How to Maintain a Healthy Body and Relationship

It is advisable to make your decision about trying to change your body weight with your doctor's help. Never trust anything you read online regarding health and weight loss. Losing weight is not recommended for everyone, and it doesn't necessarily translate into better health. It's important to remember that maintaining excellent health calls for a lifetime commitment that includes not only healthy habits but also a positive body image.

Chapter 10: Exercise and Weight Loss

Exercise's Benefits for Weight Loss

Being overweight can be bad for your health in addition to making you feel uncomfortable. According to the Centers for Disease Control and Prevention (CDC), obesity rates have skyrocketed in the US in recent years. As of 2010, obesity was defined as affecting more than one-third of Americans with a body mass index (BMI) of 30 or above. Body mass is calculated by dividing weight in pounds by height in inches by 2, then multiplying the result by 703 (weight (lb) / [height (in)] 2). The following three steps can help you calculate your body mass:

Add 703 pounds to your current weight.
the square inches of your height.
Multiply the result by one after subtracting the step 1 result from the step 3 result.

Obesity can lead to several serious health problems, including heart disease, diabetes, stroke, and numerous types of cancer.

One method for helping someone lose weight is to restrict the number of calories they eat through food. Increasing calorie burn through exercise is one alternative.

benefits of exercise over dieting
Calorie restriction alone is less effective for weight loss than a healthier diet and regular exercise. Exercise can prevent or even reverse the effects of several diseases. Exercise lowers blood pressure and cholesterol, which may help prevent a heart attack.

Exercise also lowers your risk of developing certain cancers, including breast and colon cancer. Exercise has a reputation for boosting self-esteem and general well-being, possibly lowering anxiety and depression symptoms.

Exercise helps people maintain and lose weight. Exercise can increase metabolism, which is the daily caloric expenditure rate. Lean body mass can be preserved and even grown, which raises daily caloric expenditure.

How Much Exercise Is Necessary for Weight Loss?

If you wish to reap the health advantages of exercise, it is recommended that you perform some form of aerobic activity at least three times per week for a minimum of 20 minutes per session. It's preferable to exercise for more than 20 minutes if you want to lose weight. As long as you don't consume too many calories thereafter, a daily practice of just 15 minutes of moderate exercises, such as walking a mile, can result in a 100-calorie calorie burn. 700 calories burned each week for a year can lead to a 10-pound weight loss.

How to Calculate Your Target Heart Rate

To fully benefit from exercise's health benefits, you must do some higher-intensity activities. To gauge how hard you are working, you can take your heart rate. The simplest way to get your ideal heart rate is to subtract your age from 220 and divide the result by between 60 and 80 percent.

Consult a trainer or your medical team to determine your appropriate intensity for each session. Anyone with specific health issues, such as an accident, diabetes, or a heart ailment, should consult a doctor before beginning any fitness program.

What Are Some Examples of the Different Exercise Forms?
It matters less how you exercise for weight loss than if you exercise at all. To maintain a regular schedule, experts advise picking exercises you enjoy.

Aerobic
Any fitness program you want to do must include some form of aerobic or cardiovascular exercise. The heart rate and blood circulation are

raised during aerobic exercise. Cycling, swimming, dancing, walking, and jogging are examples of aerobic exercises. You can work out with a fitness machine like a treadmill, elliptical, or stair stepper.

Training in Strength
Gaining muscle while working out with weights has various advantages, including assisting in fat loss. Muscle also burns calories. What a good feedback loop! Experts recommend doing out three times a week on all major muscle groups. This includes:

abs

back

biceps

calves

chest

forearms

hamstrings

quads

shoulders

traps

triceps

Yoga

Yoga, albeit less intense than other forms of exercise, can nonetheless aid in weight loss in a variety of ways. The study found that those who practice yoga have a lower risk of being overweight because they are more mindful of their eating habits.

Including exercise in your daily routine
The total amount of activity you get in a day is more significant than whether or not you

exercise in a specific session. As a result, even minor changes to your daily routine can significantly affect your waistline.

A healthy lifestyle consists of the following:

Using the stairs instead of the elevator, parking further away from destinations, and then walking the entire distance when running errands
the calories expended by various activities
The ordinary adult male who does not exercise needs roughly 2,200 calories per day to maintain his weight. A girl needs around 1,800 calories per day to stay at her current weight.

Following is a list of typical activities and an estimation of how many calories they burn each hour.

Activities

Calories Used

either participating in baseball, golf, or laundry

240 to 300

dancing, cycling, or other intense activity

370 to 460

walking (at a nine-minute-mile pace) (at a nine-minute-mile pace) you might go swimming or play football.

580 to 730

Skiing, racquetball, or running (at a seven-minute-mile pace)

740 to 920

Consult your doctor before starting a new exercise routine, especially if you plan to perform strenuous activities. This is especially important if you have:

cardiac condition

lung disease

diabetes

kidney disease and arthritis

People who have recently been particularly sedentary, who are overweight, or who recently gave up smoking should also speak with their doctors before starting a new fitness plan.

When you first start a new workout regimen, it's important to pay heed to your body's indications. To improve your level of fitness, you should work harder. But pushing yourself past your limits could be harmful. Stop exercising if you start to experience pain or start to get out of breath.

Chapter 11: Get outside to burn calories

The following strategies can help with weight loss when we spend more time in nature:

1. Reduce the amount of time we spend sitting.

Screen-based activities lengthen our inactive time. In front of a screen, any task is typically carried out while seated. Before you know it, you've been glued to a screen all day and into the evening. How does that make you feel physical? Mentally? Probably not good. After a demanding, inactive day, people frequently discover that eating fatty or sugary snacks can momentarily improve their mood and is the only source of physical relaxation. Sadly, they make you gain weight as well.

Mobility is a requirement for the bulk of outdoor activities, including walking the dog, biking, raking leaves, gardening, transporting kids to school, and doing errands.

2. Lessen our levels of stress.

The research is clear-cut. Even in suburban yards and urban parks, spending time in a natural environment causes your body to produce less cortisol and lower blood pressure (stress hormone). Additionally, our nerve system's calm-controlling region is more active (the parasympathetic nervous system). You can also gain this benefit by keeping plants indoors or by looking out the window at a beautiful natural setting.

Since stress is one of the biggest triggers for overeating, anything that helps to relieve stress healthily is a terrific way to stop it.

3. Make connections between us and the area.

Sadly, in some communities, residents hardly even know their neighbors. Obesity's "sleeper" causes are isolation and loneliness. People usually overlook the factors that contribute to their weight issues when thinking about them. Spending more time outside, even for just a daily 15-minute walk around your neighborhood, may help you interact with people better.

In the future, who knows how this will impact other things? I remember starting to go for everyday walks in my own life (alone). One of my neighbors noticed me from her window and came over. then another, then still another. We grew to five individuals very rapidly. Because several of us had young children, we all went for walks five days a week with them strapped in strollers. I made several new friends, and because we all enjoyed the opportunity to mingle, our brief stroll turned into a much longer one.

Every step you take outside of your door, according to the theory, brings you one step closer to leading a conscious life.

4. Develop a calm, focused attitude.

For screen time, one needs the mental capacities of "directed attention" or "voluntary attention." To complete your professional obligations, read your emails, reply to texts, and participate in all the other ways we "screen time," you must consistently put in this kind of effort. This level of concentration drains a lot of resources and finally causes mental fatigue. Despite the persistent pull of off-task thinking, attention must be kept.

When you are effortlessly involved in a task (the "flow" state), or when you are engaged in more free-form activities like strolling, jogging, thinking, or gardening, you are engaging in "involuntary attention." In contrast to the earlier, this.

Studies have been conducted to determine whether spending time in natural settings might assist us to overcome cognitive fatigue. The results demonstrated that we can. Spending time outside in the sunshine, clean air, and the presence of the sounds of nature is like pressing the reset button on our neurological system.

Our lives can become more conscious the more often we can temporarily attain this condition. This mindfulness can then be used to be conscious of our routines and eating practices.

5. Help us develop a more thorough understanding of our position within the ecosystem.

As we become more awake, we start to perceive beyond simply ourselves. Food is only one factor in how much we weigh; we are more than just our weight. On our journey toward awareness, it is not just about us. Our families, our neighborhoods, and the entire planet are affected.

We might have consumed a Chilean apple. In that single mouthful, we make connections with a farmer on another continent. Our choices have an impact on him and his family. A drought or natural disaster in another region affects us in America.

When we spend most of our time indoors, watching nature on a television screen, and hardly ever feeling the sun on our faces, it is easy to forget that we are all connected. This is not just a tired cliché. This will appear more genuine to us the more time we spend outside and away from screens.

Chapter 12: Ways to Track the Progress of Your Weight Loss

Obesity is one of the most significant health issues of our time. It contributes to a wide range of potentially fatal diseases, including but not limited to diabetes, heart issues, rheumatoid arthritis, and hypertension. Some medical experts claim that obesity raises a person's risk of getting cancer. However, people nowadays are better informed than they were ten years ago, and it seems that keeping active and healthy is getting more and more popular.

It's more important to lose weight for your health than just to look better. This path to healthy weight loss can get easier for you if you effectively track your weight loss progress. Below, I provide you with the top five ways to accomplish this.

Action Plan, first

Whatever the person's goal, making a plan is the first and one of the most important steps. Therefore, acquiring a weight loss planner is the initial step. Write the responses to the following three questions on the first page of your planner: Do you require weight loss? Why is losing weight required? What would you do to lose weight? Because many people develop an image of themselves that is consistent with the beauty standards that are common in their surroundings, the first question is important. They don't care what their healthy weight is or whether they need to reduce weight to conform to social expectations. Social acceptance shouldn't come before your health. For instance, if you are obese or have another health issue as a result of being overweight, you should take weight loss seriously. This answers the first two questions.

The last question concerns your weight-loss strategy. Think about the kind of food you would pick and the type of workout program you would set up for yourself. Your weekly or monthly diet plan might be written down in your daily planner. Additionally, to support your efforts, note helpful weight reduction suggestions in your planner. You could also document your weekly exercise schedule. Create a plan for losing weight, get a daily planner, and keep track of your results.

2. Calculation of Weight

Using a reliable body scale, you can monitor your weight daily or once a week. There are many different types of body scales available on the market. To keep things simple, we urge you to buy a digital one. It will be easier to reduce measurement error if you weigh yourself at the same time each day, at the end of each week, or every three days. Then calculate the weights' average. You should record the average in your weight loss planner. Weigh yourself before eating breakfast. You should ideally just be weighing yourself while wearing your underwear. Some people check their weight several times a day. We suggest weighing oneself every three days. Establish a particular time each day for this. Never weigh yourself after eating a meal. Don't let a weight increase or drop demotivate you because other aspects of health and fitness are just as important.

3. Important Percentages & Ratios

Numerous factors influence your weight. Your genetics, bone mass, muscle mass, body fat, water composition, age, and body mass index all play a role in determining your present weight and optimal weight (BMI). BMI is the ratio of your weight to height and serves as a gauge for what your ideal weight should be concerning your height. Your BMI can be calculated using a publicly available online BMI calculator or a fitness app. But because it completely ignores muscle mass, it shouldn't be seen in isolation. Even though many wrestlers, athletes, and bodybuilders have extraordinarily high muscle mass, their BMI alone can classify them as obese. Body fat is the proportion of fat in your body. While measuring it with vernier calipers yourself won't be perfect but will offer you a broad idea, you might try to calculate yours correctly with the help of an expert. By dividing your body weight by your body fat percentage, you may use that number to calculate your muscle mass. Ideal charts for body fat and muscle mass compositions are easily accessible online and in several apps. If you include all of these in your daily planner, you can check them again after a month. Remember that these are factors that should be considered simultaneously and that they will change over time.

4. Body Measurements

You can learn more about your development from regular body measures than from weight checks alone. The ratios and percentages discussed above are essential, but some of them are difficult to calculate and others even require spending money. The easiest and cheapest option is to get one inch of tape and take measurements with it. The most important measurement to take while keeping track of your growth is the circumference of your waist, but you should also measure other body parts including your chest, biceps, forearms, thighs, and waist. Measure them once a week, ideally before breakfast. Make sure you measure them precisely.

A fifth point is Mirror, Mirror on the Wall.
Standing in front of a full-length mirror in nothing but your underwear, take a photo with your phone. Although it may seem ludicrous, this is one of the best and simplest ways to detect physical improvements in yourself while exercising and dieting. Take a photo every 15 days. The date would be automatically captured by your camera. For your privacy, you can save these pictures in a different folder and use folder lock software to lock them with a password. To obtain the best indication of your progress, try dressing in the tightest items in your wardrobe and take a picture every 15 days.

www.ingramcontent.com/pod-product-compliance
Lightning Source LLC
Chambersburg PA
CBHW050828250726
48653CB00006B/2482